TABLE CONTENTS

Chapter 1

Introduction

In the intricate tapestry of our daily lives, health and vitality stand as the threads that weave our experiences together. Yet, amid the complexities of modern living, we often overlook the profound impact our habits have on our well-being. Welcome to "Alkaline Habits: The Key to Balance and Wellness," a transformative exploration into the fundamental principles of harmonious living and holistic health.

A. Definition of Alkaline Habits

At the heart of this journey lies the concept of alkaline habits, a lifestyle centered around nurturing our bodies with alkaline-forming choices. But what exactly are alkaline habits? These are the deliberate, conscious choices we make each day, designed to maintain the body's natural alkaline state. Through mindful decisions in our diet, hydration, exercise, and overall lifestyle, we can tip the scales towards alkalinity, promoting a balanced internal environment that fosters health and vitality.

B. Importance of pH Balance in the Body

Central to our understanding is the pH balance within our bodies—an intricate equilibrium that dictates our overall health. The pH scale, ranging from acidic to alkaline, measures the balance of hydrogen ions in our system. Maintaining an optimal pH balance is not merely a biological function; it is the cornerstone of vibrant health. In this e-book, we delve deep into the science behind pH balance, unraveling its importance in every bodily function and illuminating the profound impact it has on our energy, immunity, and longevity.

C. The Impact of Alkaline Habits on Overall Health

As we explore the impact of alkaline habits, we will uncover their far-reaching effects on our holistic well-being. From bolstering our immune system to enhancing mental clarity, these habits serve as the catalyst for transformative change. By embracing alkaline choices, we provide our bodies with the optimal environment to thrive, fostering a sense of vitality that radiates from within.

D. Preview of Alkaline Lifestyle Benefits

Embarking on the path of alkaline habits opens the door to a myriad of benefits, each more transformative than the last. In this e-book, we will preview the tangible advantages of an alkaline lifestyle. From increased energy levels that fuel your passions to a strengthened immune system that shields you from illnesses, you will witness the tangible rewards that come with embracing this holistic approach to living.

Join us on this enlightening journey through the realm of alkaline habits. As we navigate the nuances of pH balance, unravel the intricacies of holistic health, and preview the bountiful benefits of an alkaline lifestyle, you will embark on a profound transformation—one that transcends the physical and touches the very essence of your being. Your path to balance, vitality, and wellness starts here. Let's begin this empowering voyage together.

Chapter 2

Understanding pH Balance

In the intricate symphony of our bodies, maintaining the delicate balance of pH is akin to composing a harmonious melody. In this chapter, we will journey through the fundamental concepts of pH balance, unraveling the mysteries of acidity and alkalinity, and understanding how this balance profoundly influences our overall well-being.

A. Explanation of the pH Scale

At the heart of understanding pH balance lies the pH scale, a numerical scale ranging from 0 to 14. The pH scale measures the acidity or alkalinity of a solution, with 7 being neutral. Solutions with a pH less than 7 are acidic, while those with a pH greater than 7 are alkaline. This chapter will provide you with a comprehensive insight into this scale, empowering you to decipher the pH levels of various substances, including the foods you consume and the beverages you drink.

B. Alkaline vs. Acidic: Balancing Act

Life is a delicate balance between alkalinity and acidity. While some acidic elements are essential for bodily functions, excessive acidity can disrupt this balance and lead to various health issues. Conversely, embracing alkaline choices in your diet and lifestyle acts as a counterbalance, restoring equilibrium within. We will explore the importance of this balancing act, guiding you on how to make mindful choices that promote alkalinity and maintain the crucial balance between acidic and alkaline elements in your body.

C. How pH Balance Affects Various Body Functions

PH balance plays a pivotal role in every aspect of our physiology. From the digestive system, where it influences enzyme activity and nutrient absorption, to the immune system, where it affects the body's ability to ward off infections, understanding pH balance is key to unlocking optimal health. In this section, we will delve into the intricate ways pH balance impacts various bodily functions, shedding light on how a balanced pH fosters efficient cellular processes and overall wellness.

D. Common Misconceptions about Alkalinity

As we journey deeper into the realm of pH balance, it is essential to dispel common misconceptions that often shroud the concept of alkalinity. Misinformation can hinder progress toward adopting alkaline habits. This section will address prevalent myths and misconceptions, equipping you with accurate knowledge and empowering you to make informed decisions about your lifestyle choices.

By the end of this chapter, you will not only have a clear understanding of the pH scale but also appreciate the significance of maintaining a balanced pH in your body. Armed with this knowledge, you will be better prepared to embrace the transformative power of alkaline habits, laying the foundation for a healthier, more vibrant you. Stay tuned as we delve even deeper into the practical applications of this understanding in the chapters that follow, guiding you toward a life brimming with balance and vitality.

Chapter 3

The Alkaline Diet

In this chapter, we embark on a culinary adventure, exploring the transformative power of the alkaline diet. Here, we will uncover the essence of this nourishing lifestyle, learn to differentiate between alkaline and acidic foods, master the art of creating alkaline balance in every meal, and dive into a world of tantalizing alkaline recipes and meal plans.

A. What is the alkaline diet?

The Alkaline Diet is not merely a meal plan; it's a philosophy of mindful eating. At its core, the alkaline diet emphasizes consuming foods that promote an alkaline environment within the body. By focusing on fresh fruits, vegetables, legumes, nuts, and seeds and minimizing acidic choices such as processed foods, dairy, and refined sugars, this diet aims to maintain the body's natural pH balance. In this section, we will delve into the principles that underpin the alkaline diet, providing you with a solid foundation to embark on this transformative culinary journey.

B. Alkaline Foods vs. Acidic Foods

Understanding the distinction between alkaline and acidic foods is key to implementing the alkaline diet effectively. We will explore an extensive list of alkaline and acidic foods, empowering you to make informed choices. By comprehending the impact of different foods on your body's pH levels, you will be equipped with the knowledge to craft meals that support alkalinity, leading to enhanced energy levels and overall well-being.

C. Creating Alkaline Balance in Meals

Creating alkaline balance in your meals involves more than just choosing the right foods. It's about crafting well-balanced, flavorful dishes that not only nourish your body but also delight your taste buds. In this section, we will uncover practical strategies for combining alkaline ingredients creatively. From incorporating diverse textures and colors to experimenting with various cooking methods, you will learn the art of constructing satisfying, alkaline-balanced meals that are as visually appealing as they are delicious.

D. Alkaline Recipes and Meal Plans

Prepare to tantalize your senses with a collection of delectable alkaline recipes and meal plans carefully curated to support your journey toward optimal health. From vibrant salads and refreshing smoothies to hearty main courses and guilt-free desserts, these recipes showcase the versatility of alkaline ingredients. Additionally, we will provide you with sample meal plans, guiding you through a day of alkaline eating and ensuring that you never feel deprived while embracing this transformative lifestyle.

As you delve into the culinary delights of the alkaline diet, you will not only nourish your body but also awaken your taste buds to a world of flavors that support your overall well-being. With the knowledge and recipes provided in this chapter, you will be well on your way to embracing the alkaline diet with confidence and enthusiasm, propelling yourself further along the path to a healthier, more balanced life. Bon appétit!

Chapter 4

Alkaline Hydration

In this section, we delve into the vital realm of alkaline hydration, exploring the profound significance of staying properly hydrated for maintaining pH balance within the body. We will uncover the benefits and sources of alkaline water, learn how to create alkaline water at home, and explore a delightful array of other alkaline beverages, including teas, smoothies, and juices.

A. Importance of Hydration in maintaining pH Balance

Hydration is the cornerstone of a healthy body, and it plays a pivotal role in maintaining optimal pH balance. We will unravel the connection between hydration and pH balance, understanding how adequate water intake supports cellular functions, enhances detoxification, and fosters an alkaline environment within. By appreciating the crucial link between hydration and pH balance, you will be empowered to make informed choices to support your body's natural equilibrium.

B. Alkaline Water: Benefits and Sources

Alkaline water stands as a beacon of hydration excellence, offering benefits beyond regular water. In this section, we explore the unique advantages of alkaline water, from its enhanced hydration capabilities to its potential antioxidant properties. We will also discuss various sources of alkaline water, guiding you on how to choose the best options available on the market to align with your alkaline lifestyle.

C. DO IT YOURSELF Alkaline Water Recipes

Why buy alkaline water when you can create your own? This segment unveils the secrets behind crafting your personalized alkaline water at home. With simple ingredients and easy-to-follow recipes, you can elevate your hydration game and ensure a constant supply of fresh, alkaline-rich water. We will provide you with step-by-step instructions, allowing you to experiment with different flavors and find the perfect alkaline water recipe that suits your taste buds and health goals.

Recipe 1: Lemon Alkaline Water

Ingredients:

- 1 lemon, sliced
- 1-2 liters of purified water

Instructions:

1. Fill a pitcher with 1-2 liters of purified water.
2. Add the sliced lemon to the water.
3. Let the mixture sit for 1-2 hours before drinking to allow the lemon's alkalizing properties to infuse into the water.
4. Enjoy your homemade lemon alkaline water!

Recipe 2: Cucumber Mint Alkaline Water

Ingredients:

- 1/2 cucumber, thinly sliced
- a handful of fresh mint leaves
- 1-2 liters of purified water

Instructions:

1. Add cucumber slices and fresh mint leaves to a pitcher.
2. Pour 1-2 liters of purified water into the pitcher.
3. Let the mixture infuse in the refrigerator for at least 2-4 hours or overnight.
4. Strain out the cucumber and mint leaves, and your cucumber and mint alkaline water is ready to be served.

Recipe 3: Berry Alkaline Water

Ingredients:

- 1 cup mixed berries (such as strawberries, blueberries, and raspberries)
- 1-2 liters of purified water

Instructions:

1. Mash the mixed berries slightly with a fork to release their juices.
2. Place the mashed berries in a pitcher.
3. Pour 1-2 liters of purified water into the pitcher.
4. Let the mixture steep in the refrigerator for a few hours or overnight.
5. Strain out the berry solids, and your refreshing berry alkaline water is ready to drink.

Recipe 4: Herbal Alkaline Water

Ingredients:

- A few sprigs of fresh herbs (such as basil, rosemary, or thyme)
- 1-2 liters of purified water

Instructions:

1. Crush the fresh herbs gently to release their flavors.
2. Add the crushed herbs to a pitcher.
3. Pour 1-2 liters of purified water into the pitcher.
4. Allow the mixture to infuse for at least 2-4 hours or overnight in the refrigerator.
5. Strain out the herbs, and your herbal-infused alkaline water is ready to be served.

Remember to use fresh, organic ingredients for the best results. Experiment with different fruits, vegetables, and herbs to create your own unique alkaline water recipes tailored to your taste preferences. Enjoy your homemade alkaline water while staying hydrated and healthy!

D. Other Alkaline Beverages: Teas, Smoothies, and Juices

Alkaline hydration isn't limited to water alone. In this part of the chapter, we will explore a delightful variety of alkaline beverages. From revitalizing teas infused with herbs and fruits to nutrient-packed smoothies that serve as complete meals and refreshing juices bursting with vitamins and minerals, we will guide you through the creation of these beverages. Each recipe not only quenches your thirst but also contributes to maintaining your body's pH balance, ensuring you stay refreshed, energized, and alkaline throughout the day.

With the knowledge gained from this chapter, you will not only understand the significance of alkaline hydration but also be equipped with practical skills to create a diverse range of alkaline beverages tailored to your preferences. Let's raise a glass to your health and alkalinity! Cheers!

Chapter 5

Alkaline Habits for Physical Health

In this section, we explore a multifaceted approach to physical health through alkaline habits. By aligning your exercise routine, skincare practices, sleep patterns, and supplement choices with alkalinity, you can enhance your overall well-being and vitality.

A. Alkaline Exercise

Optimal Workouts for pH Balance Exercise is not just about burning calories; it's a fundamental aspect of maintaining pH balance and holistic health. In this chapter, we delve into the world of alkaline exercises, guiding you through routines that promote pH balance. From yoga and Pilates to aerobic exercises, you'll discover how specific workouts can support your body's alkaline state, providing you with energy, flexibility, and strength. Learn how to tailor your exercise regimen to not only keep you fit but also to enhance your body's natural alkalinity.

EXERCISE AND THE ALKALINE LIFESTYLE

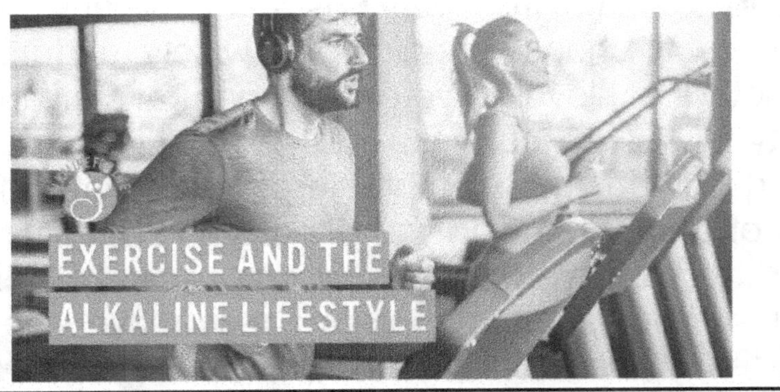

B. Alkaline Skin Care

Natural Beauty Routines Your skin, the body's largest organ, deserves the best care possible. In this part of the chapter, we focus on alkaline skincare routines that harness the power of natural ingredients. Explore the benefits of alkaline cleansers, moisturizers, and masks, and learn how to create your own skincare products using alkaline-forming elements. By nurturing your skin with alkaline care, you can achieve a radiant complexion while supporting your body's overall pH balance.

C. Alkaline Sleep

Importance of Rest and Recovery Sleep is the body's ultimate healer, essential for both physical and mental well-being. In this section, we emphasize the importance of alkaline sleep patterns. We discuss the impact of rest on pH balance and explore ways to improve the quality of your sleep naturally. Discover relaxation techniques, bedtime rituals, and sleep environment adjustments that promote alkalinity, allowing you to wake up refreshed, rejuvenated, and ready to face the day.

D. Alkaline Health Supplements

Making Informed Choices Supplements can complement your diet and support your body's alkaline balance. However, not all supplements are created equal. In this chapter, we provide a comprehensive guide to alkaline health supplements, from vitamins and minerals to herbal remedies. Learn how to choose supplements wisely, understanding their impact on your body's pH levels. We explore natural supplements that promote alkalinity, ensuring you make informed choices to bolster your overall health and well-being. By embracing alkaline habits for physical health, you are not only enhancing your fitness and beauty but also nurturing your body in a way that aligns with its natural alkaline state. Through optimal workouts, natural skincare, restorative sleep, and mindful supplement choices, you can cultivate physical vitality and radiance that emanate from within. Your journey to physical well-being starts here. Let's embrace these alkaline habits together, nurturing your body in harmony with nature.

Chapter 6

Alkaline Mindset and Emotional Well-Being

In this section, we delve into the profound connection between your mindset, emotional well-being, and alkaline living. By addressing stress, incorporating mindfulness practices, nurturing positive relationships, and embracing habits that enhance mental clarity and focus, you can create a resilient and alkaline mindset that fosters inner harmony and emotional balance.

A. Stress and Its Impact on pH Balance

Stress, often a silent intruder in our lives, can significantly disrupt our body's pH balance. This chapter begins by unraveling the intricate relationship between stress and pH balance. Understanding how stress affects your body's alkalinity is the first step toward managing it effectively. We explore stress-reducing techniques and holistic approaches that not only alleviate stress but also contribute to a more alkaline internal environment.

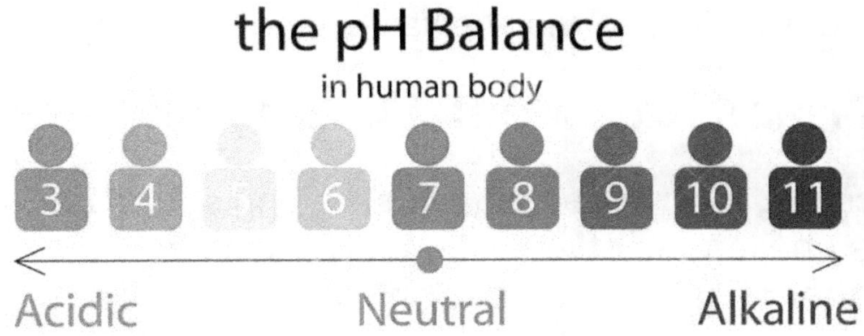

B. Alkaline Mindfulness: Meditation and Relaxation Techniques

Mindfulness is a powerful tool that anchors you to the present moment, reducing anxiety and promoting emotional equilibrium. Here, we dive into the world of alkaline mindfulness, exploring meditation and relaxation techniques tailored to support your alkaline lifestyle. From guided meditation to mindful breathing exercises, you will learn practical strategies to enhance your mental well-being, balance your emotions, and maintain your body's optimal pH levels.

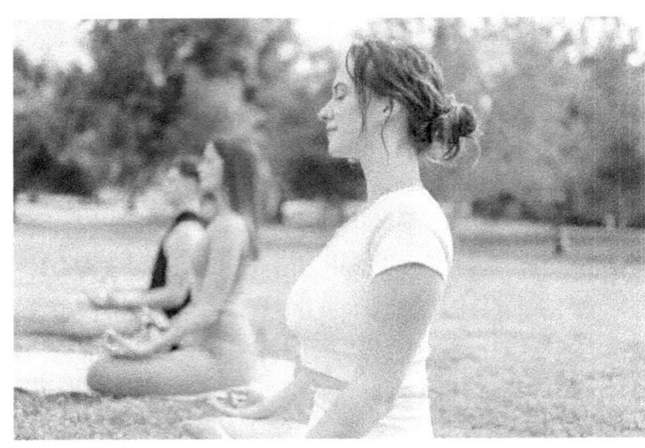

C. Cultivating Positive Relationships for Alkaline Living

Our relationships profoundly impact our emotional state and overall well-being. In this part of the chapter, we focus on the importance of cultivating positive relationships for alkaline living. We explore effective communication, empathy, and conflict resolution strategies that nurture healthy connections. Positive relationships not only support emotional well-being but also contribute to a more alkaline and harmonious lifestyle.

D. Alkaline Habits for Mental Clarity and Focus

A clear and focused mind is essential for making sound decisions and navigating life's challenges effectively. In this section, we explore specific alkaline habits that enhance mental clarity and focus. From nutrition and hydration to sleep patterns and exercise routines, you will discover how these habits impact your cognitive functions. Implementing these habits in your daily life can sharpen your mind, improve your concentration, and promote overall mental acuity.

By adopting an alkaline mindset and embracing practices that enhance emotional well-being, you can transform the way you perceive and respond to life's challenges. Through stress management, mindfulness techniques, positive relationships, and habits that foster mental clarity, you will cultivate an alkaline mindset that empowers you to navigate life with grace and resilience. Your emotional well-being is a vital aspect of your alkaline journey, and by embracing these practices, you are nurturing a positive and alkaline mind that forms the foundation for a vibrant and balanced life.

Chapter 7

Overcoming Challenges

In this section, we address the hurdles commonly faced when transitioning to an alkaline lifestyle. By understanding these challenges and implementing effective strategies, you can overcome resistance, navigate temptations, find inspiration in real-life success stories, and sustain your alkaline habits in the long run.

A. Common Challenges in Adopting Alkaline Habits

Embarking on an alkaline journey is transformative, yet it's not without its challenges. This chapter begins by identifying the most common obstacles faced when adopting alkaline habits. From social pressures to cravings for acidic foods, we shed light on these challenges, providing you with a clear understanding of what to expect on your alkaline journey.

B. Strategies for Overcoming Resistance and Temptations

Resisting temptations and overcoming resistance is crucial for maintaining consistency in your alkaline habits. In this section, we explore effective strategies to tackle these challenges head-on. From mindful decision-making to building a support system, you will learn practical techniques to stay on track, even in the face of the most tempting acidic indulgences.

C. Success Stories: Real-life Examples of Alkaline Transformation

Inspiration is a powerful motivator. In this part of the chapter, we present real-life success stories of individuals who have transformed their lives through alkaline habits. These stories showcase the tangible benefits of embracing an alkaline lifestyle, from increased energy levels and weight loss to improved overall health. Reading about the triumphs of others will empower you, demonstrating that your goals are not only achievable but also within reach.

D. Tips for Sustaining Alkaline Habits in the Long Run

Sustainability is the key to long-term success. In this final section, we provide you with invaluable tips for sustaining your alkaline habits in the long run. From creating a personalized support network to incorporating alkaline habits into your daily routines, you will receive practical advice to ensure that your alkaline lifestyle becomes a permanent and integral part of your life.

By acknowledging common challenges, implementing effective strategies, drawing inspiration from real-life successes, and adopting sustainable practices, you can overcome obstacles and establish a strong foundation for your alkaline habits. Armed with the knowledge and motivation provided in this chapter, you will not only conquer challenges but also thrive, making alkaline living an enduring and rewarding part of your journey to optimal health and well-being. Remember, every challenge overcome is a step closer to a vibrant and alkaline you. Stay resilient, stay inspired, and let your alkaline journey transform your life.

Chapter 8

Alkaline Habits for Environmental Sustainability

In this chapter, we explore the symbiotic relationship between alkaline habits and environmental sustainability. By adopting eco-friendly practices, making sustainable dietary choices, reducing exposure to environmental toxins, and understanding the global impact of our habits, we can contribute to a healthier planet while enhancing our own well-being.

A. Alkaline Habits and Eco-Friendly Practices

The choices we make in our daily lives have a direct impact on the environment. In this section, we examine how alkaline habits align with eco-friendly practices. From reducing plastic waste to conserving energy and water, you will learn how embracing an alkaline lifestyle can contribute to a greener, more sustainable planet. Discover practical tips to minimize your ecological footprint and make a positive impact on the environment.

B. Sustainable Eating: Alkaline Choices for the Planet

The food we consume plays a significant role in environmental sustainability. Here, we explore the concept of sustainable eating within the framework of an alkaline diet. Learn about locally sourced produce, organic farming, and seasonal eating habits that support both your health and the planet. By making mindful choices about the food you consume, you can promote sustainable agricultural practices and contribute to a more eco-conscious world.

C. Reducing Environmental Toxins for Alkaline Living

Environmental toxins can disrupt the body's natural balance and affect overall well-being. In this part of the chapter, we focus on reducing exposure to environmental toxins to support alkaline living. Explore natural cleaning products, eco-friendly personal care items, and toxin-free home environments. By minimizing your exposure to harmful substances, you not only safeguard your health but also contribute to a cleaner, healthier planet.

D. Alkaline Habits and Global Environmental Impact

Our individual actions, when multiplied across the globe, have a profound impact on the environment. In this final section, we zoom out to examine the global environmental impact of our collective alkaline habits. Discover how small changes in our daily routines can create a ripple effect, influencing industries and policies. By being mindful of our choices and advocating for environmentally conscious practices, we can be catalysts for positive change on a global scale.

By incorporating eco-friendly practices, making sustainable dietary choices, reducing exposure to environmental toxins, and understanding the global impact of our habits, we can align our alkaline lifestyle with environmental sustainability. By nurturing a harmonious relationship with the planet, you not only enhance your own well-being but also contribute to a healthier, more balanced world for generations to come. Embrace these alkaline habits with a sense of purpose, knowing that your choices are not only transforming your life but also making a positive difference for the Earth.

Chapter 9

Alkaline Habits and Disease Prevention

In this chapter. Alkaline habits refer to adopting a lifestyle centered around consuming alkaline-forming foods and maintaining an alkaline-acidic balance in the body. These habits focus on incorporating a diet rich in fruits, vegetables, nuts, seeds, and whole grains, which are alkaline in nature. The idea behind alkaline habits is to reduce the body's acidic load, which proponents believe can contribute to various health benefits, including disease prevention.

Disease prevention, in the context of alkaline habits, refers to the proactive approach of using alkaline diets and lifestyle choices to reduce the risk of chronic illnesses and other health conditions. While scientific research on the direct relationship between alkaline diets and disease prevention is still evolving, proponents claim that maintaining an alkaline environment in the body can help prevent diseases such as heart disease, diabetes, cancer, and osteoporosis. These claims are often based on the belief that an acidic internal environment can create conditions conducive to the development and progression of various diseases. Alkaline habits are aimed at counteracting this acidity by consuming foods that promote alkalinity, which, according to some theories, can support overall health and well-being. It's important to note that the efficacy of these practices and their direct impact on disease prevention are areas of ongoing research and debate within the scientific community.

A. Alkalinity and Chronic Disease

The relationship between alkalinity and chronic disease prevention has been a subject of increasing interest in the scientific community. Maintaining optimal alkalinity in the body through a balanced diet rich in alkaline foods such as fruits, vegetables, and whole grains is thought to have potential benefits for preventing chronic diseases. Chronic inflammation, a common denominator in many chronic diseases, is believed to be mitigated by alkaline diets. By creating an alkaline environment, these habits might help reduce the risk of diseases such as heart disease, diabetes, and arthritis. Research suggests that an alkaline diet can counterbalance the acidic load in the body, potentially offering a protective effect against various chronic ailments.

B. Alkaline Habits for Heart Health

Alkaline habits play a pivotal role in nurturing heart health. An alkaline diet, primarily comprising fresh fruits, vegetables, nuts, and seeds, is abundant in heart-friendly nutrients like potassium and magnesium. These elements are crucial in regulating blood pressure and maintaining heart rhythm. Additionally, alkaline-rich foods are often low in cholesterol and saturated fats, making them heart-healthy choices. By promoting a balanced pH level and reducing inflammation, alkaline habits contribute to arterial health, potentially reducing the risk of heart diseases, including hypertension and atherosclerosis. The alkaline lifestyle supports cardiovascular well-being, acting as a preventive measure against heart-related issues.

C. Alkaline Living and Cancer Prevention

Alkaline living, characterized by an emphasis on alkaline-forming foods, holds promise in the realm of cancer prevention. The link between an acidic environment in the body and the proliferation of cancer cells has spurred interest in alkaline diets as a potential preventive measure. Alkaline-rich foods, notably leafy greens, cruciferous vegetables, and citrus fruits, are replete with antioxidants and phytonutrients. These compounds are believed to neutralize harmful free radicals, reducing the risk of cellular mutations that can lead to cancer. Moreover, by fostering an alkaline pH balance, these habits create an unfavorable environment for cancer cell growth. While more research is needed, adopting an alkaline lifestyle with a focus on plant-based, nutrient-dense foods may play a role in cancer prevention strategies, offering a proactive approach to overall health and well-being.

D. Alkaline Habits for Diabetes Management and Prevention

Alkaline habits can play a role in diabetes management and prevention by promoting a balanced diet, maintaining a healthy weight, and improving overall well-being. While these habits are not a cure for diabetes, they can be part of a holistic approach to managing the condition and reducing the risk of developing type 2 diabetes. Here are some ways alkaline habits can contribute to diabetes management and prevention:

1. **Balanced Diet:** Alkaline diets emphasize whole, nutrient-dense foods such as fruits, vegetables, nuts, and seeds. These foods are low in processed sugars and unhealthy fats, promoting stable blood sugar levels. Consuming a balanced diet can help regulate glucose levels, which is essential for managing diabetes and reducing the risk of developing the condition.
2. **Weight Management:** Maintaining a healthy weight is crucial for diabetes management and prevention. Alkaline diets, which often include low-calorie, high-fiber foods, can support weight loss and help prevent obesity. Excess weight, especially around the abdomen, is a significant risk factor for type 2 diabetes. Alkaline habits can contribute to achieving and maintaining a healthy weight.
3. **Reducing Inflammation:** Chronic inflammation is associated with insulin resistance, a key factor in type 2 diabetes. Alkaline-rich foods, particularly fruits and vegetables, are anti-inflammatory and can help reduce inflammation in the body. By lowering inflammation, alkaline habits may contribute to improving insulin sensitivity.
4. **Enhancing Insulin Sensitivity:** Some studies suggest that alkaline diets can improve insulin sensitivity, allowing the body to use insulin more effectively. This can be beneficial for individuals with insulin resistance, a common precursor to type 2 diabetes. Improved insulin sensitivity means better control of blood sugar levels.
5. **Promoting Hydration:** Alkaline water, which has a higher pH level than regular water, is often included in alkaline diets. Staying well-hydrated is essential for overall health and can help regulate blood sugar levels. Proper hydration supports kidney function, which is important for individuals with diabetes.
6. **Encouraging Physical Activity:** Alkaline habits are often complemented by an active lifestyle. Regular exercise is beneficial for managing diabetes as it helps lower blood sugar levels and improve insulin sensitivity. Combining alkaline habits with physical activity can enhance the overall impact on diabetes management and prevention.

It's important to note that individual responses to dietary changes vary, and consulting a healthcare provider or a registered dietitian is crucial before making significant changes to one's diet, especially for individuals with diabetes or those at risk of developing the condition. Personalized guidance can help create an appropriate and effective diabetes management plan tailored to individual needs and health goals.

Chapter 10

Conclusion

In this final chapter, we bring our alkaline journey to a close, summarizing the transformative principles of alkaline habits. Reflect on the benefits, find encouragement to continue your journey, and embrace a call to action to implement alkaline habits today. Additionally, discover a wealth of resources and references for further reading to support your ongoing exploration of this alkaline lifestyle.

A. Recap of Alkaline Habits and Their Benefits

Let's revisit the fundamental aspects of alkaline habits. We've explored pH balance, the alkaline diet, hydration, physical health, mindset, and environmental sustainability. By incorporating these principles into your life, you're enhancing your overall well-being, promoting vitality, and creating a balanced and alkaline you. Remember the benefits, from increased energy levels to improved mental clarity and emotional balance, and acknowledge the positive changes you've experienced.

B. Encouragement for Readers to Embrace an Alkaline Lifestyle

I want to commend you on your dedication to embracing an alkaline lifestyle. Your commitment to your health and well-being is commendable. Remember, this is a journey, not a destination. Continue to embrace alkaline habits with enthusiasm, and let your commitment fuel your progress. Believe in your ability to achieve optimal health and vibrant living.

C. Call to Action: Implementing Alkaline Habits Today

The time to act is now. Take the knowledge and inspiration from this book and put it into practice. Start implementing alkaline habits today—in your diet, exercise routine, mindfulness practices, and environmental choices. Small, consistent changes can lead to significant results over time. Take one step at a time, be patient with yourself, and celebrate your victories along the way.

As you close the pages of this book, remember that you hold the key to your well-being. Embrace the alkaline lifestyle with determination, positivity, and a thirst for knowledge. By continuing to nurture your body, mind, and spirit with alkaline habits, you are not only investing in your health but also creating a life filled with balance, vitality, and joy. Seize this opportunity, embrace the alkaline way of living, and let it guide you to a future of wellness and fulfillment. Your alkaline journey is just beginning; make it vibrant; make it yours.